A Note from the Author

If you enjoyed this book or found it helpful, I would be so grateful if you could take a moment to share your thoughts. Reviews not only support my work but also help others discover resources that may benefit their own wellness journey.

✦ Leave a review on Amazon:
This book was created with AI assistance. While effort has been made to ensure accuracy, the content is for informational purposes only.

★ Or share your feedback on Google:
This book was created with AI assistance. While effort has been made to ensure accuracy, the content is for informational purposes only.

Thank you for being part of the Empower Your Wellness community! Your support means so much.

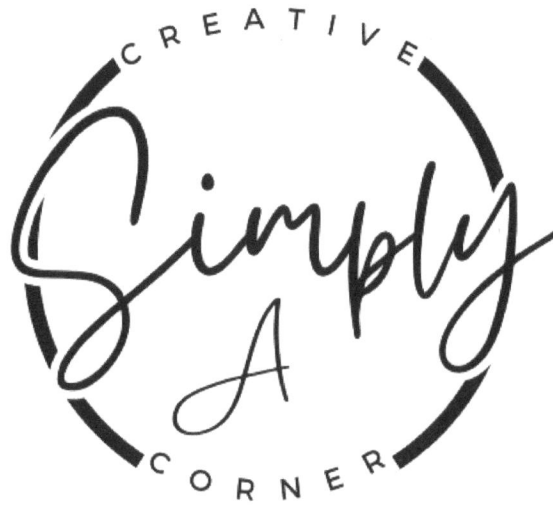

"Welcome to "Herb and Spice Mastery: A Beginner's Comprehensive Guide"! We are delighted to have you embark on this enlightening journey with us. While we may not be experts, we are enthusiastic learners, just like you. Our exploration of the realm of herbs and spices began in the spring of 2023, offering both challenges and rich rewards.

This ebook series was crafted to serve as a complete resource, covering everything you need to know about each herb and spice. Whether you seek quick facts, detailed insights into cultivation, or practical uses, we've got you covered. Remember, we always advise consulting a physician before using any herb or spice for medicinal purposes.

As we progress and acquire more knowledge, we are thrilled to share our discoveries with you through new ebooks. Each edition delves into a different herb, spice, or medicinal plant, expanding our shared knowledge and enriching our well-being together.

Thank you for joining us on this expedition. We hope you derive as much joy and value from these pages as we did in creating them. Let's learn and progress together!"

TABLE OF
CONTENTS

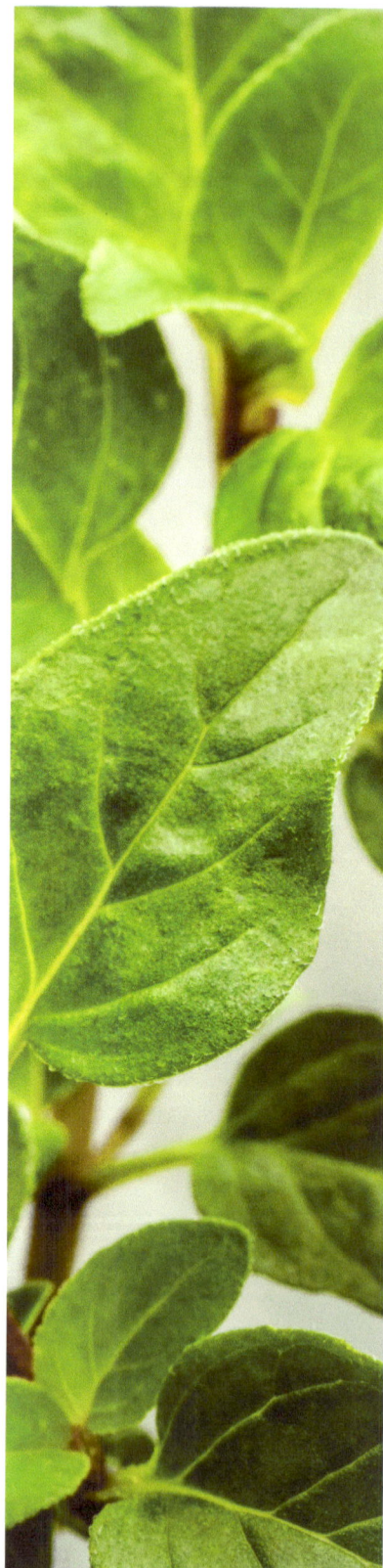

BRIEF HISTORY

The use of Eucalyptus plants at home for health benefits has a rich history rooted in ancient herbal traditions. Indigenous Australians were pioneers in utilizing Eucalyptus for its medicinal properties, using it for wound care, fever relief, and respiratory health. They crushed the leaves to make healing poultices or inhaled the steam to clear congestion. This knowledge later influenced early settlers and spread globally.

When Eucalyptus oil became commercially available in the 19th century, its popularity surged, especially for home remedies. Many households began using Eucalyptus oil for its antiseptic properties, applying it to cuts or burns and using it to freshen the air or deter pests. In the Victorian era, it was common for people to grow small Eucalyptus plants on patios or in conservatories to access fresh leaves and enjoy their invigorating scent, which was believed to purify indoor air.

Today, the trend of growing Eucalyptus at home has returned, especially for its benefits in natural health and wellness. Its leaves can be used in teas, bath soaks, and essential oils to support respiratory health, improve mood, and promote relaxation. Eucalyptus plants are not only valued for their practical health benefits but also for adding a touch of nature indoors.

Eucalyptus trees, while native to Australia, are adaptable and can grow in a variety of climates worldwide. Here are some regions outside Australia where Eucalyptus thrives:

Mediterranean Climates: Eucalyptus has been successfully introduced to Mediterranean regions, including parts of southern Europe (Spain, Portugal, Italy) and North Africa. The warm, dry summers and mild, wet winters suit many Eucalyptus species.

Africa: Eucalyptus trees grow extensively in East Africa (Ethiopia, Kenya, and South Africa) and are valued for timber, fuel, and erosion control.

South America: Eucalyptus plantations are common in Brazil, Argentina, and Uruguay. Brazil, in particular, has vast Eucalyptus forests grown for timber and pulp industries due to the rapid growth rate in the warm climate.

North America: Certain species of Eucalyptus can grow in parts of California and Florida. The mild climates of these regions allow Eucalyptus to thrive, especially for ornamental use and windbreaks.

Asia: Eucalyptus is also grown in India and China. In India, it's particularly valued for its timber and oil production and grows well in states with warmer climates, like Kerala and Tamil Nadu.

Our focus on Eucalyptus stems from its significant therapeutic value, particularly for respiratory health, skin care, and as a natural insect repellent. Known for its essential oils, which have powerful antimicrobial, anti-inflammatory, and decongestant properties, Eucalyptus has become a staple in natural remedies and modern wellness. This ebook aims to explore the full potential of Eucalyptus, guiding readers from seed to usage, allowing them to understand and harness its benefits responsibly and effectively.

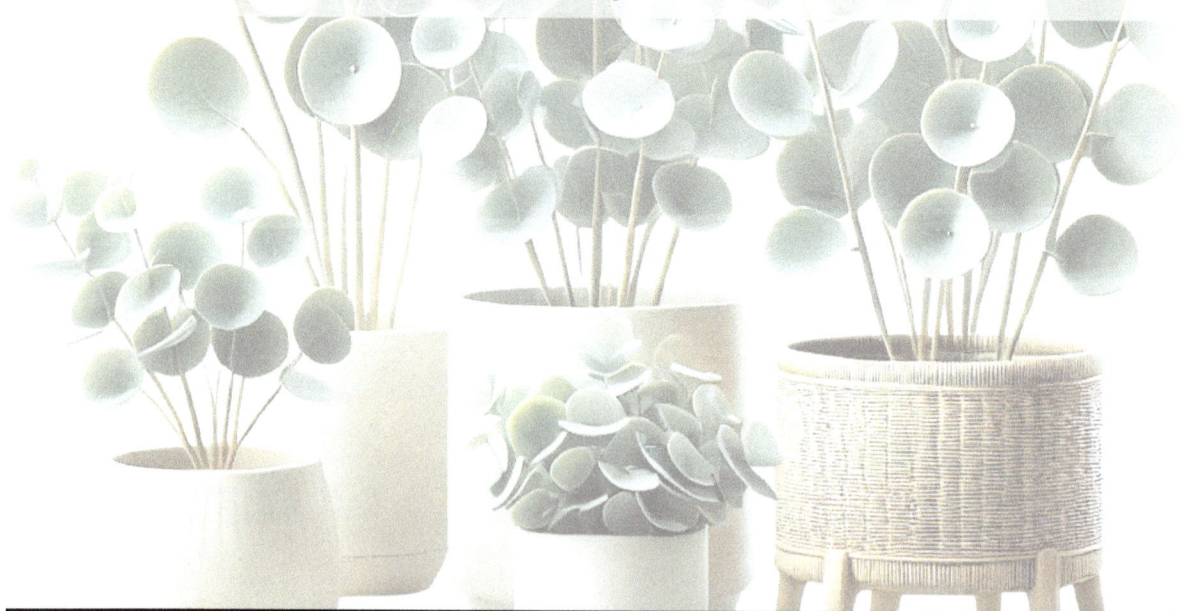

A

LEGAL NAME
Eucalyptus

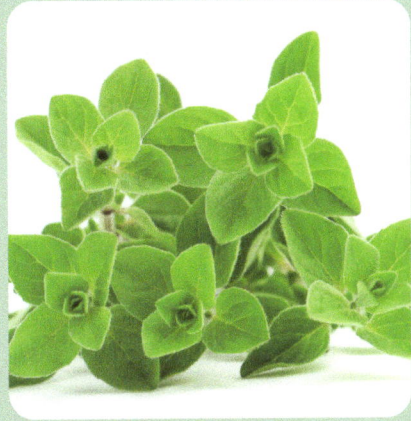

B

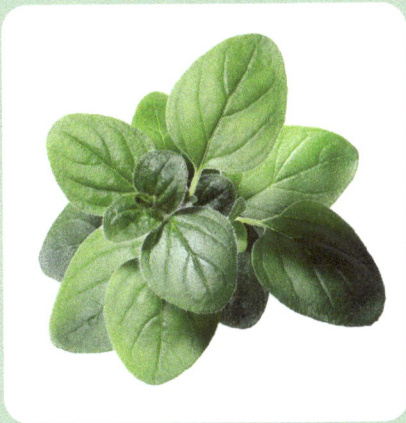

FAMILY.
Myrtoideae

C

BOTANICAL

Eucalyptus is an evergreen tree or shrub with smooth, peeling bark and aromatic blue green leaves. It has uniquee flowers without petals, featuring fluffy, colorful stamens, and produces woody capsula shaped fuits called gumnuts that release seeds when mature.

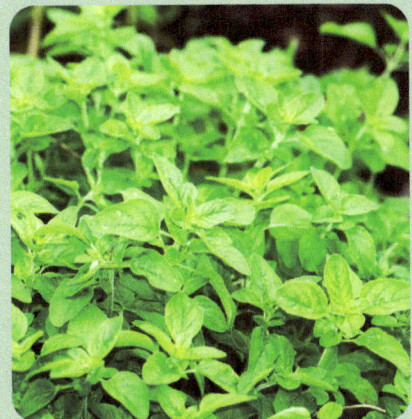

Health & Medicinal Benefits

The medicinal components in the Eucalyptus plant include various active compounds that contribute to its health benefits. Here are the primary ones:

1 Eucalyptol (Cineole):

This is the main compound in eucalyptus oil, comprising up to 90% of its composition. Eucalyptol is a powerful decongestant, anti-inflammatory, and antimicrobial agent, making it effective for respiratory relief, pain reduction, and fighting infections.

2 Flavonoids:

These are antioxidants found in the leaves, which help reduce oxidative stress in the body. The primary flavonoids in eucalyptus include quercetin, rutin, and catechin, which support the immune system and may reduce inflammation.

3 Tannins:

Eucalyptus leaves contain tannins, which have astringent properties that can aid in wound healing by constricting tissue and reducing minor bleeding. They also have anti-inflammatory effects, contributing to skin and wound care.

4 Terpenes:

Compounds such as alpha-pinene, limonene, and globulol contribute to the plant's antimicrobial and anti-inflammatory effects. Terpenes are also responsible for the plant's distinctive aroma and enhance the overall therapeutic benefits in essential oil form.

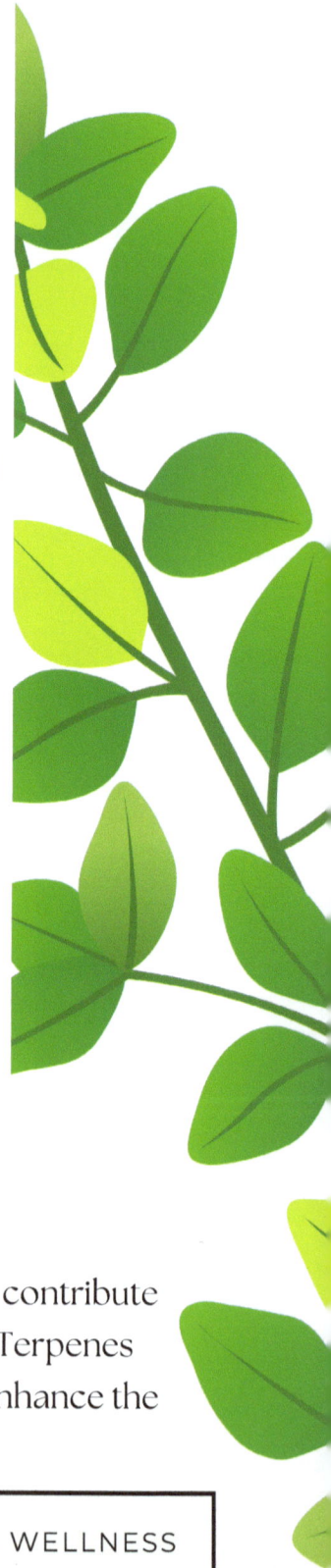

5 Phenolic Acids:

Compounds like chlorogenic acid and caffeic acid in eucalyptus have antioxidant and anti-inflammatory properties, supporting cardiovascular health and general immune function.

Health Benefits

Eucalyptus offers a variety of health and medicinal benefits, primarily through its essential oil, which contains compounds like eucalyptol (cineole) known for their therapeutic properties:

1 Respiratory Health

Eucalyptus is widely used for respiratory issues, as it acts as a natural decongestant and helps relieve symptoms of coughs, colds, asthma, and bronchitis. Inhalation of eucalyptus vapors or steam therapy can ease congestion and soothe inflamed airways.

2 Antimicrobial and Antiseptic

Eucalyptus oil has strong antimicrobial properties, making it effective for wound care and infection prevention. It is often used in natural disinfectants, mouthwashes, and skin products for its ability to kill bacteria, fungi, and viruses.

3 Pain Relief and Anti-Inflammatory

Eucalyptus can help reduce muscle pain, joint inflammation, and arthritis discomfort due to its anti-inflammatory and analgesic properties. Topical application of diluted eucalyptus oil can alleviate sore muscles and promote relaxation.

4 Mental Clarity and Relaxation

The fresh, invigorating scent of eucalyptus promotes mental clarity and relieves stress. Aromatherapy with eucalyptus is known to boost mood, relieve fatigue, and improve focus.

5 Insect Repellent

Eucalyptus oil is a natural insect repellent and can keep mosquitoes and other pests at bay. It's often used in outdoor sprays and lotions for its effectiveness in deterring bugs.

These components make eucalyptus a potent plant for health uses, especially for respiratory, skin, and muscle relief.

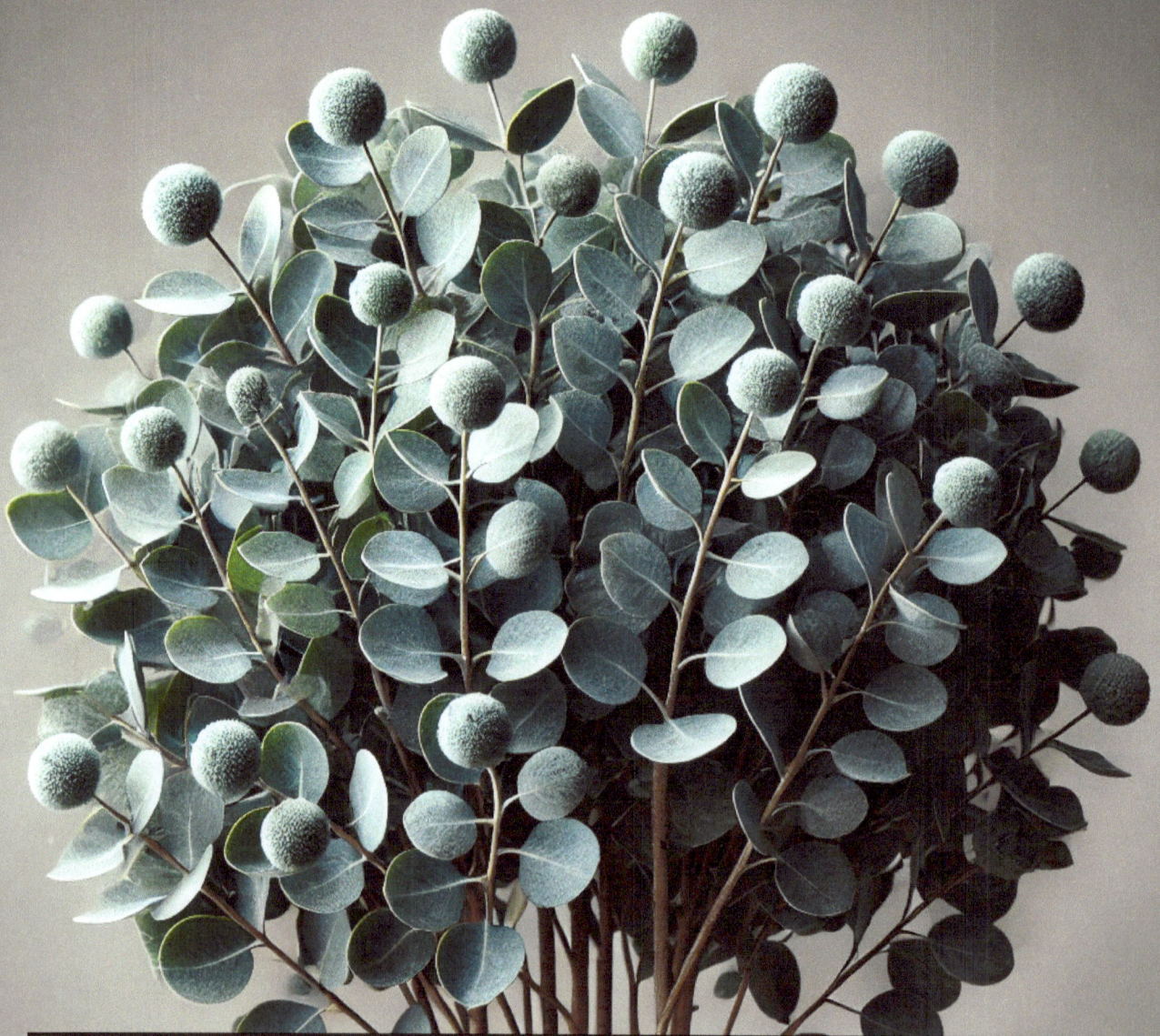

Preparations & Uses & Dosages

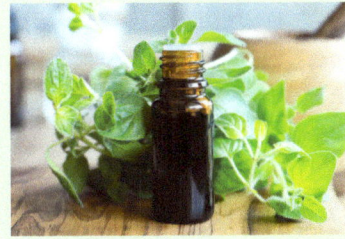

01   Eucalyptus Steam Inhalation (For Respiratory Relief)

- Ingredients:
    - 5–10 fresh or dried eucalyptus leaves (or 5 drops eucalyptus essential oil)
    - Bowl of boiling water
- Instructions:
    a. Place the eucalyptus leaves in a bowl and pour boiling water over them.
    b. Lean over the bowl, covering your head with a towel to trap steam.
    c. Inhale deeply for 5–10 minutes to relieve congestion.
- Use: Helps clear nasal passages and relieve symptoms of colds, sinusitis, and bronchitis.

02   Eucalyptus Oil Chest Rub (For Coughs and Colds

- Ingredients:
    - 1/4 cup coconut or olive oil
    - 10 drops eucalyptus essential oil
- Instructions:
    a. Melt coconut oil if solid, and mix with eucalyptus oil.
    b. Allow the mixture to cool and solidify in a small container.
    c. Rub a small amount onto the chest and throat before bedtime.
- Use: Provides a warming effect to ease breathing and soothe coughs.

03   Eucalyptus Tea (For Immune Support)
- Ingredients:
  - 1–2 fresh or dried eucalyptus leaves
  - 1 cup boiling water
- Instructions:
  - a. Rinse the leaves and tear them slightly to release oils.
  - b. Place the leaves in a cup and pour boiling water over them.
  - c. Steep for 5–10 minutes, then strain.
  - d. Sweeten with honey if desired.
- Use: Helps soothe sore throats, reduce inflammation, and support immune health. Avoid excessive consumption.

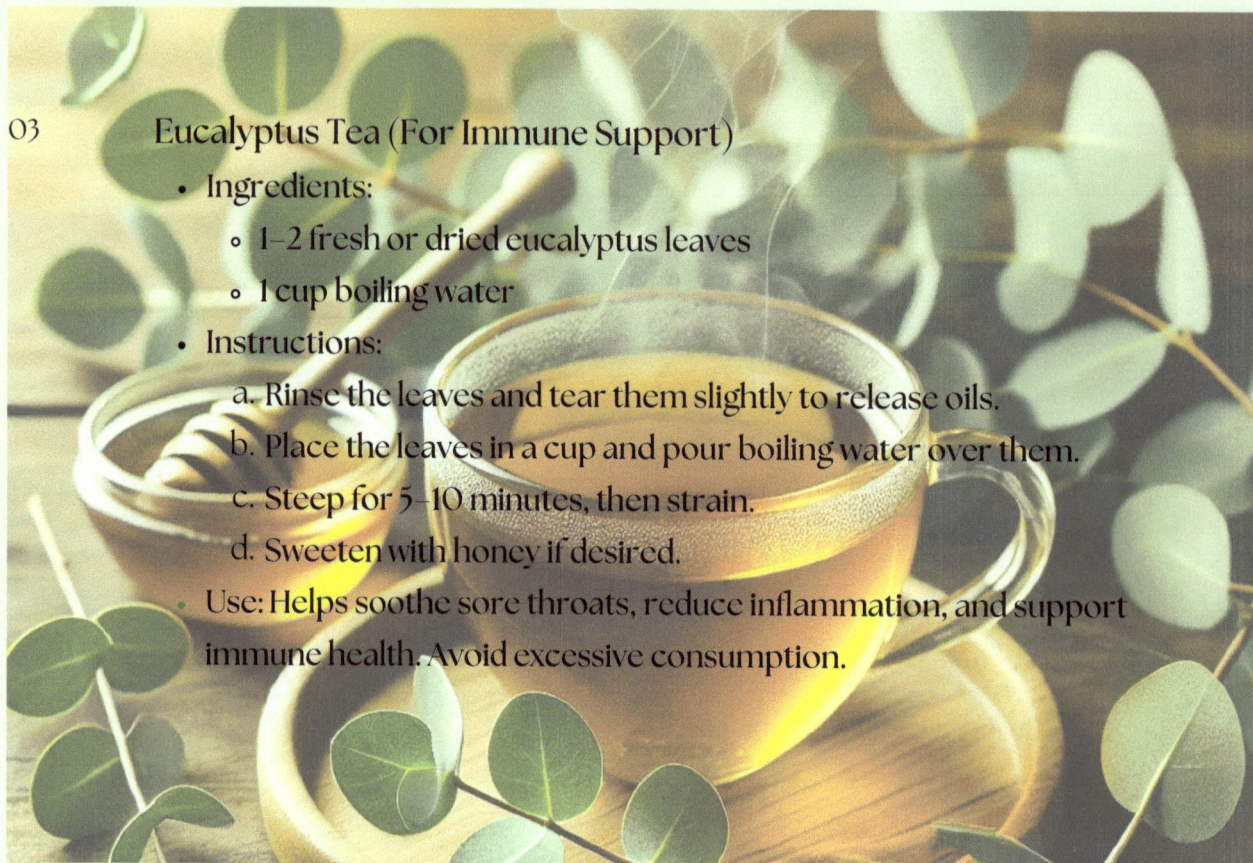

04   Eucalyptus Infused Oil (For Muscle Relief)
- Ingredients:
  - 1/2 cup carrier oil (olive, almond, or coconut oil)
  - Fresh eucalyptus leaves (enough to loosely fill a jar)
- Instructions:
  - a. Fill a jar with eucalyptus leaves, then pour carrier oil over them to cover.
  - b. Close the jar and store in a warm, sunny spot for 2–3 weeks, shaking occasionally.
  - c. Strain the oil and store it in a clean bottle.
- Use: Apply as a massage oil for sore muscles and joints, or add a few drops to bath water for relaxation.

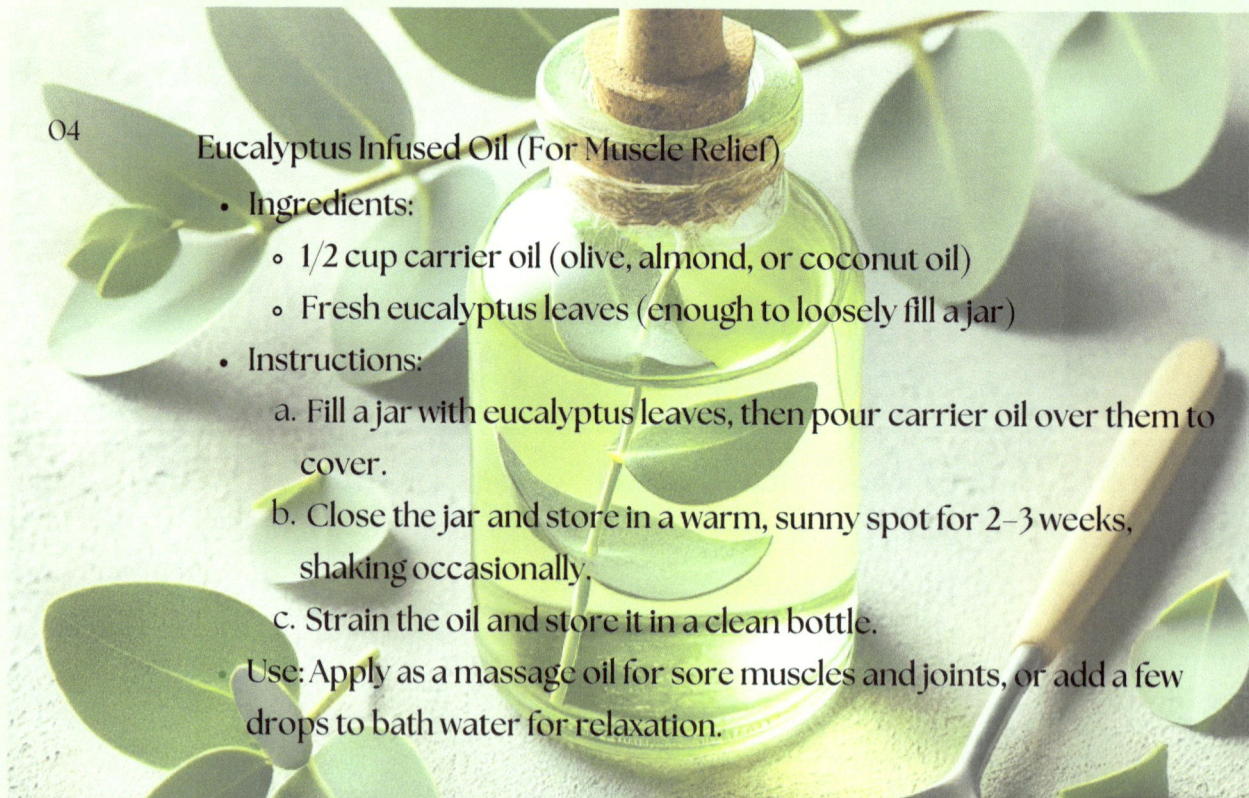

05   Eucalyptus Salve (For Pain Relief)

- Ingredients:
  - 1/4 cup eucalyptus-infused oil (see above)
  - 1 tablespoon beeswax
  - 5 drops eucalyptus essential oil
- Instructions:
  a. Melt beeswax in a double boiler and add eucalyptus-infused oil.
  b. Stir until combined, then add eucalyptus essential oil.
  c. Pour into a small container and let it solidify.
- Use: Rub onto sore areas to relieve muscle and joint pain.

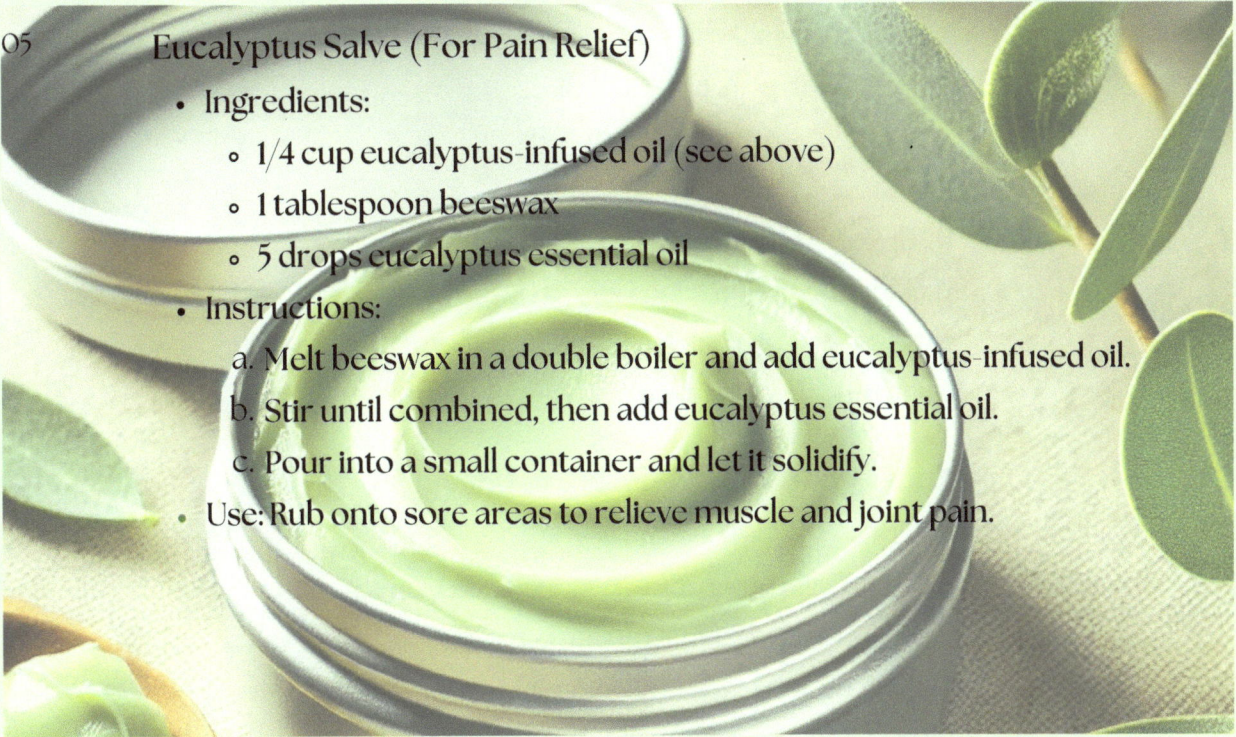

06   Eucalyptus Disinfectant Spray (Natural Cleaner)

- Ingredients:
  - 1 cup distilled water
  - 1/2 cup white vinegar
  - 15 drops eucalyptus essential oil
- Instructions:
  a. Combine water, vinegar, and eucalyptus oil in a spray bottle.
  b. Shake well before each use.
  c. Spray onto surfaces and wipe with a clean cloth.
- Use: Acts as a natural antibacterial and antiviral cleaner for household surfaces.

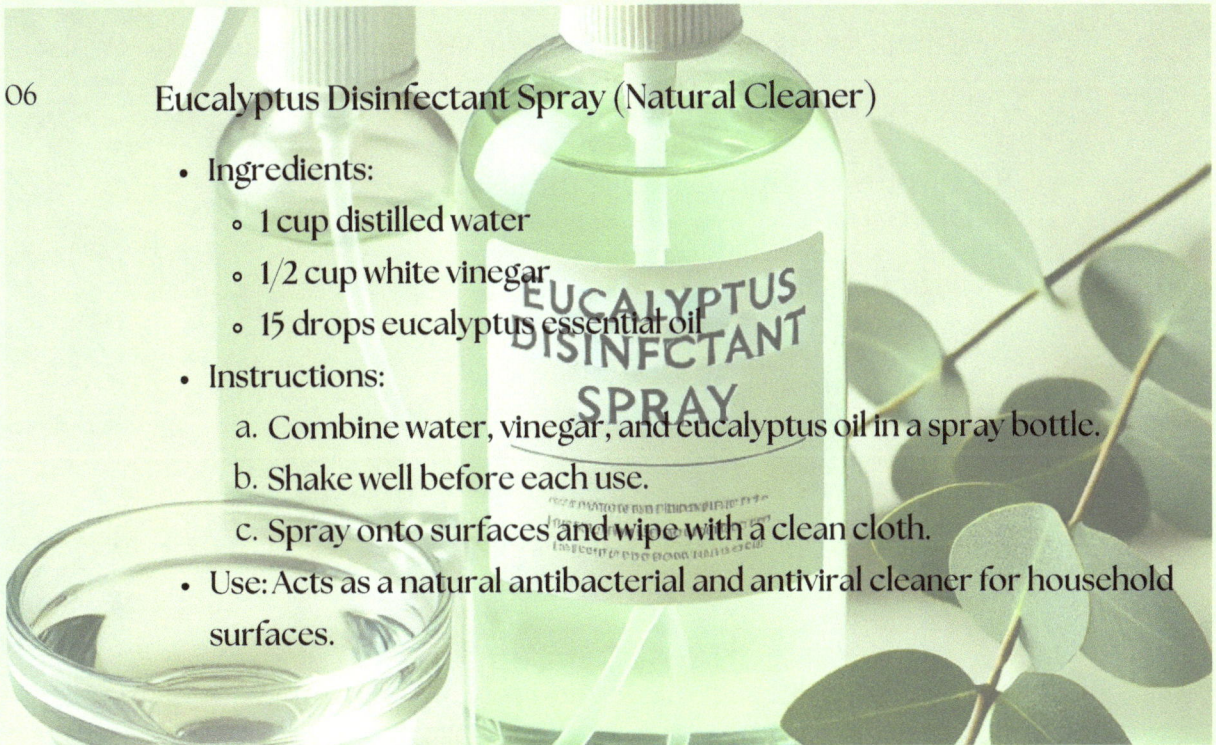

07 Eucalyptus Bath Soak (For Relaxation & Respiratory Health

- Ingredients:
    - 1/2 cup Epsom salt
    - 5 drops eucalyptus essential oil
    - Optional: Fresh eucalyptus leaves
- Instructions:
    a. Mix Epsom salt with eucalyptus oil in a bowl.
    b. Sprinkle the mixture into warm bathwater.
    c. Add fresh eucalyptus leaves for extra aroma if desired.
- Use: Eases muscle pain, clears airways, and promotes relaxation.

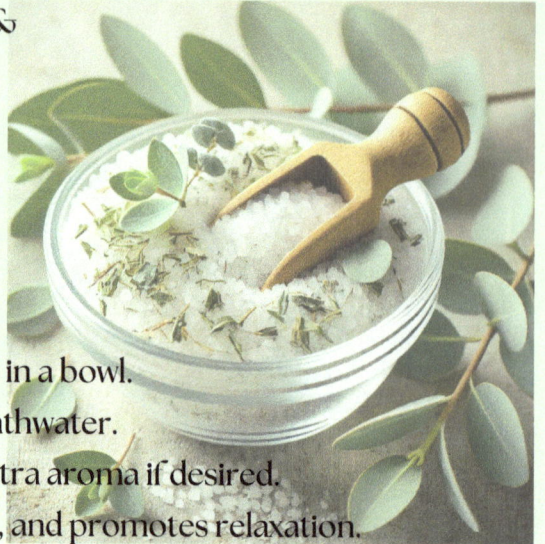

08 Eucalyptus Herbal Sachets (Insect Repellant)

- Ingredients:
    - Dried eucalyptus leaves
    - Small cloth sachets or muslin bags
- Instructions:
    a. Crush dried eucalyptus leaves and place them into small cloth sachets.
    b. Tie securely and place in closets, drawers, or under pillows.
- Use: Acts as a natural insect repellent, keeping moths and mosquitoes away.

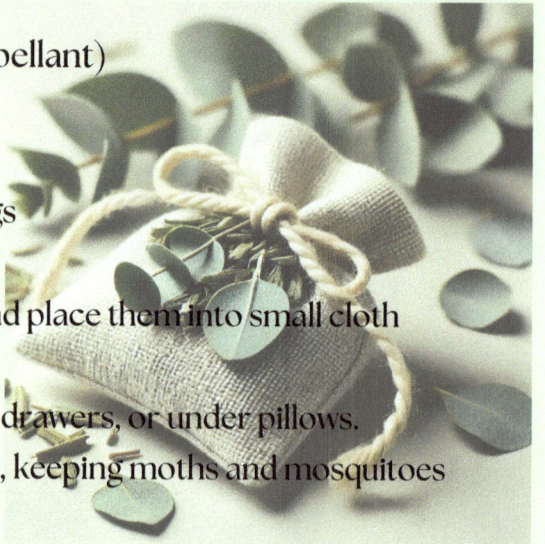

09 Eucalyptus Compress (For Wounds & Inflammation

- Ingredients:
    - 2–3 drops eucalyptus essential oil
    - Warm water
    - Clean cloth
- Instructions:
    a. Add eucalyptus oil to warm water.
    b. Soak a clean cloth in the water, wring it out, and apply it to the affected area.
- Use: Helps disinfect minor cuts and relieve inflamed skin.

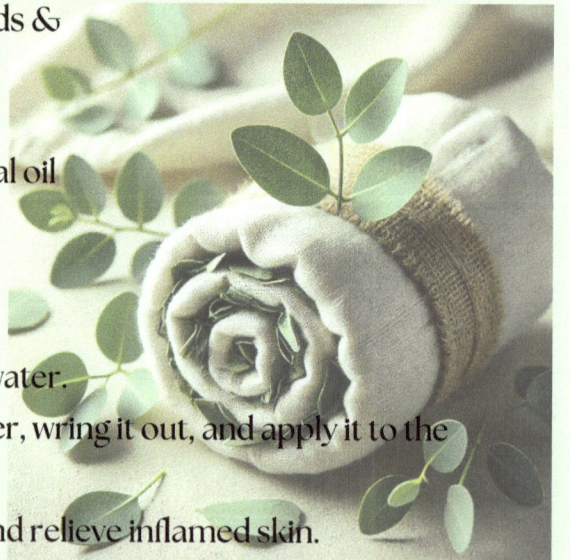

Planting

1. BEST TIME TO PLANT

Outdoors: Plant Eucalyptus seeds or young plants in spring after the last frost.
Indoors: Start seeds indoors 10–12 weeks before the last frost, typically in late winter.

3. SOWING

- Seeds: Sow eucalyptus seeds just below the soil surface and lightly cover.
- Spacing: Space seeds or young plants about 6 feet apart outdoors due to their wide spread.

Containers: Use well-draining seed-starting mix in small pots for indoor planting.

5. WATERING NEEDS

Young Plants: Maintain consistently moist soil without waterlogging; eucalyptus dislikes sitting in water.
Mature Plants: Established eucalyptus is drought-tolerant; water every 1–2 weeks in dry conditions, otherwise rely on rainfall.

2. SOIL PREPARATION

- Eucalyptus prefers well-draining, slightly acidic to neutral soil (pH 5.5–6.5).
- Amend dense soil with compost or sand for proper drainage and prevent root rot.

Avoid overly rich soils, as they can hinder growth.

4. LIGHT AND TEMPERATURE

Light: Eucalyptus thrives in full sunlight; place it outdoors in a sunny spot or by a bright south-facing window indoors.
Temperature: It prefers warm temperatures (65–75°F or 18–24°C) and is sensitive to frost; bring it indoors below 32°F (0°C).

6. SEED GERMINATION

Germination Time: Eucalyptus seeds germinate in 14–21 days at ~70°F (21°C).
Moisture: Keep soil moist but not overwatered; use a humidity dome or plastic wrap to maintain moisture.
Care After Germination: Gradually acclimate seedlings to lower humidity and direct sunlight by removing covers for longer periods daily.

Growing & *Maintenance*

01. Spacing

For outdoor planting, space eucalyptus plants 6–10 feet apart to allow for natural spreading as they mature.

For container growing, use a pot that allows at least 12 inches of root space to prevent root binding and maintain a manageable size.

02. Temperatures sunlight req

Temperature: Eucalyptus thrives in warm climates, with ideal temperatures between 65–75°F (18–24°C). They can tolerate some heat but are sensitive to frost; below 32°F (0°C), plants should be protected or brought indoors.

Sunlight: Eucalyptus requires full sun to grow optimally. Place in a spot that receives at least 6–8 hours of direct sunlight daily.

03. Soil & PH levels

Soil Type: Eucalyptus prefers well-draining, sandy or loamy soil. Heavy, clay-like soil is not suitable as it can lead to root rot.

pH Levels: Eucalyptus grows best in slightly acidic to neutral soil, with an ideal pH between 5.5 and 6.5. You can test the soil and add amendments as necessary to maintain this range.

04. Watering Needs

Young Plants: Water young eucalyptus plants regularly to keep the soil consistently moist, but avoid waterlogging.

Mature Plants: Once established, eucalyptus is relatively drought-tolerant and only needs occasional deep watering, about once every 1–2 weeks in dry conditions. In humid or rainy climates, additional watering may not be necessary.

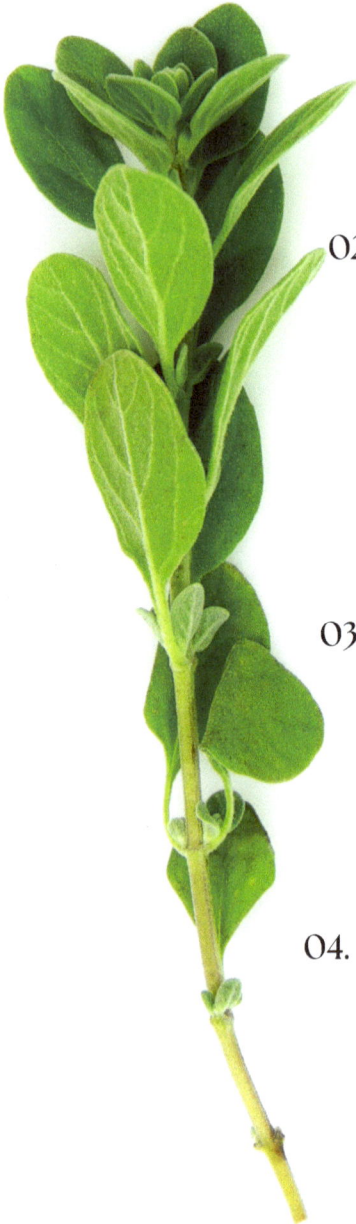

05. Care & Maintenance

Pruning: Regular pruning is essential, especially for container-grown eucalyptus, to maintain a manageable size and encourage bushier growth. Prune any dead or overgrown branches to keep the plant healthy.

Mulching: Add a layer of mulch around the base of the plant to retain soil moisture, reduce weed growth, and regulate soil temperature. Avoid piling mulch directly against the stem.

Pest Control: Eucalyptus is generally pest-resistant, but keep an eye out for pests like psyllids, which can damage the leaves. Use organic insecticidal soap if needed.

06. Fertilization

Young Plants: Eucalyptus generally does not require much fertilization, but young plants may benefit from a balanced, slow-release fertilizer (10-10-10) applied once in spring.

Established Plants: For mature eucalyptus, fertilization is often unnecessary as they are adapted to nutrient-poor soils. If growth is slow or the plant appears stressed, use a light application of balanced fertilizer during the growing season.

With these practices, your eucalyptus plants will thrive, whether grown outdoors or in containers, providing fragrant foliage and hardy greenery.

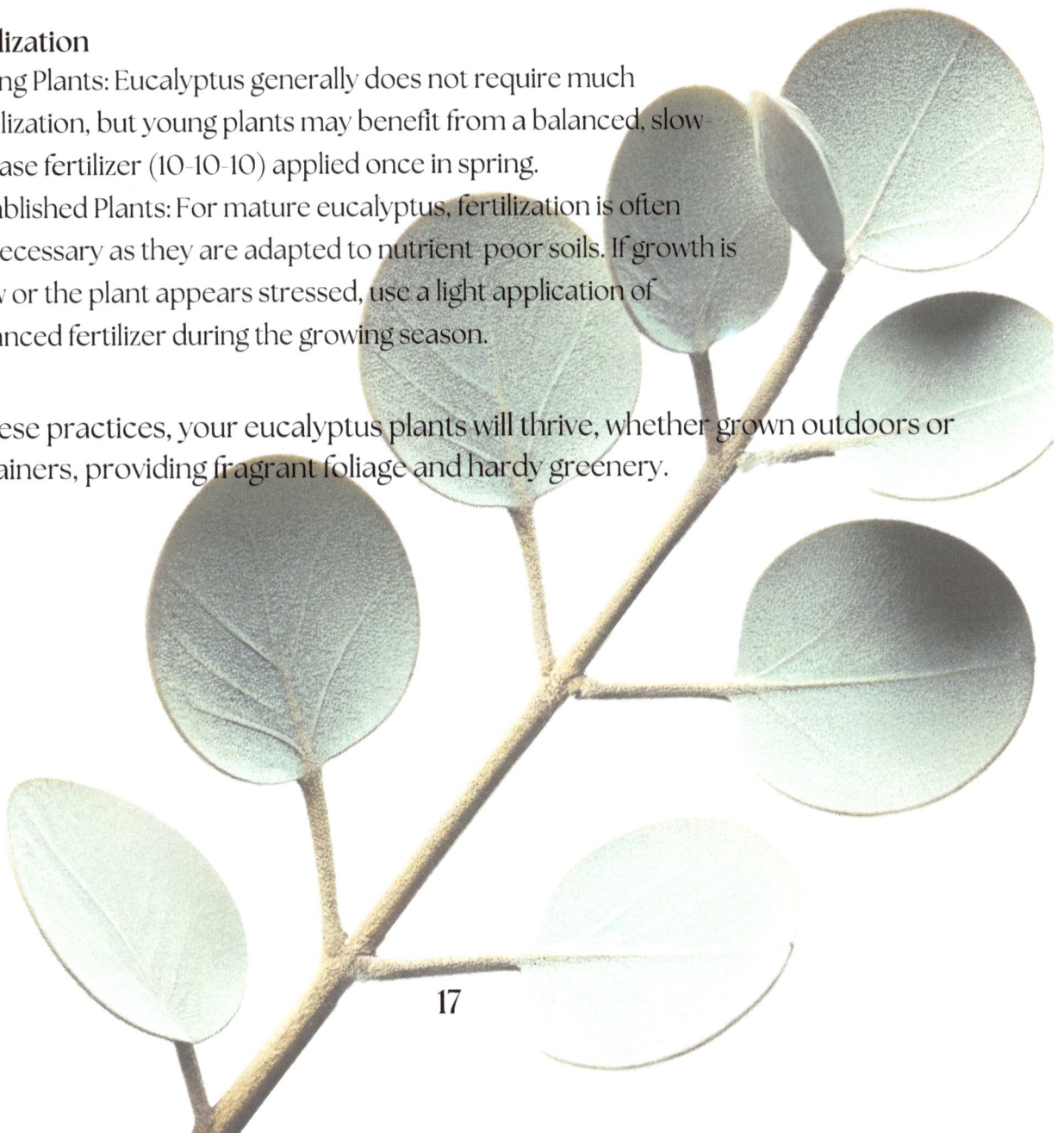

Propagation

Cuttings

Eucalyptus can be propagated from cuttings, especially younger stems that are non-woody (semi-hardwood cuttings). This method is often preferred for preserving the parent plant's specific traits. Eucalyptus cuttings require the following steps:

1. Choose a Healthy Stem from the parent plant, ideally 4–6 inches long, with a couple of leaf nodes.
2. Remove Lower Leaves and use a rooting hormone to encourage root formation.
3. Place in a Well-Draining Soil Mix and maintain high humidity to support root development.

This method typically takes a few weeks to establish roots, and it's commonly used for some varieties of eucalyptus in warmer climates.

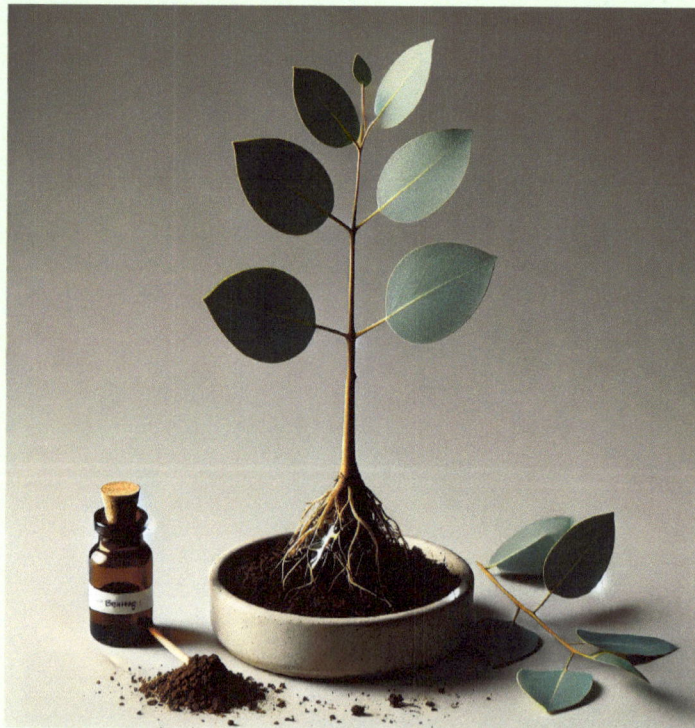

Harvesting

Harvesting eucalyptus involves gathering its leaves, stems, or branches at the right time for optimal aroma, potency, and usability. Here's a detailed guide to eucalyptus harvesting:

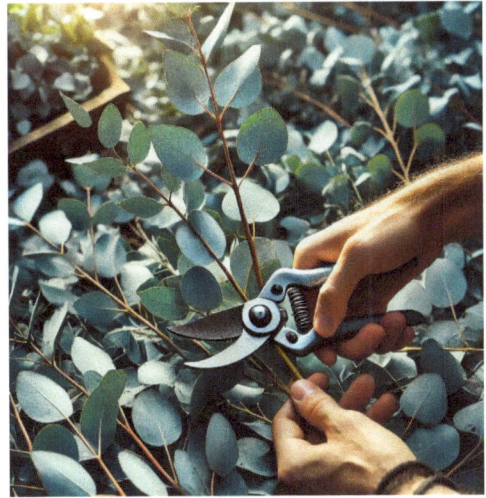

When to Harvest

Timing: The best time to harvest eucalyptus is during the late morning, after the dew has dried but before the day gets too hot. Harvesting in mid-spring to late summer yields the most potent oils, as this is when the plant's growth and oil production peak.

Maturity: Choose mature, healthy stems with fully developed leaves. Younger plants or new growth may not have as strong a fragrance or medicinal properties.

Harvesting Technique

Tools: Use clean, sharp pruning shears to prevent damaging the plant and to make a clean cut.

Method: Cut stems at an angle just above a leaf node or branching point. This encourages the plant to continue growing and helps maintain a bushier shape.

Length: Cut stems of 6–12 inches, depending on your use (e.g., smaller pieces for oils or teas, longer branches for drying and decor).

Harvesting for Essential Oil Extraction

Leaves: The leaves are the primary part harvested for oil extraction. Select mature leaves for higher oil concentration.

Quantity: Gather enough leaves for distillation, as they are dense in oil only when used in large quantities.

Storage: If not processing immediately, store the leaves in a cool, dry place out of direct sunlight to preserve oil content.

Harvesting for Fresh Use or Decoration

Leaves and Branches: For fresh bouquets, arrangements, or household use, cut longer branches with several leaves attached.

Water: Place harvested stems in water immediately to keep them fresh and prevent wilting if they are to be used for decor or fragrance.

Harvesting for Drying

Drying Method: Hang eucalyptus branches upside down in a cool, dark, and dry place with good air circulation. It can take 2–3 weeks for eucalyptus to dry completely.

Storage: Once dried, store eucalyptus in an airtight container away from light to preserve its aroma.

Frequency of Harvesting

Pruning and Regrowth: Eucalyptus responds well to regular pruning and can often be harvested multiple times a season. Leave enough foliage for the plant to regenerate, generally not removing more than one-third of the plant at a time.

Drying & *Preserving*

Drying is a transformative process, concentrating the herb's flavors and medicinal compounds, and making it shelf-stable for future use.

01 Preparation

- Choose Fresh Stems: Harvest eucalyptus stems with mature leaves, as they have a higher oil content and will retain their fragrance longer.
- Clean the Stems: Remove any damaged or brown leaves, and shake off excess dirt or debris. Trimming the stems to a uniform length can also help in the drying process.
- Optional Step: For extra fragrance, you can lightly spray the eucalyptus with a eucalyptus essential oil mist before drying.

02 Air-Drying

- Gather Stems: Bundle 4–6 stems together. Secure them with a rubber band or twine, which will tighten as the stems dry and shrink.
- Hang the Bundles: Hang the bundles upside down in a cool, dry, and dark place with good air circulation. A closet, pantry, or any low-humidity space is ideal, as high humidity can lead to mold growth.
- Drying Time: Eucalyptus usually takes 2–3 weeks to dry completely. Check periodically, ensuring the leaves feel dry and slightly brittle to the touch before removing.

03 Preserving Eucalyptus with Glycerin (Optional)

- Mix Solution: Combine two parts water to one part glycerin in a vase or container.
- Trim Stems: Cut the stems at an angle and lightly crush the bottoms to help with glycerin absorption.
- Soak the Stems: Place the eucalyptus stems upright in the solution, with the lower portion submerged. Leave them in the solution for 2–6 weeks, or until the leaves feel soft and supple.
- Drying Post-Soak: Remove the stems from the solution and let them air-dry for a few days. This process preserves the color and makes the leaves less brittle.

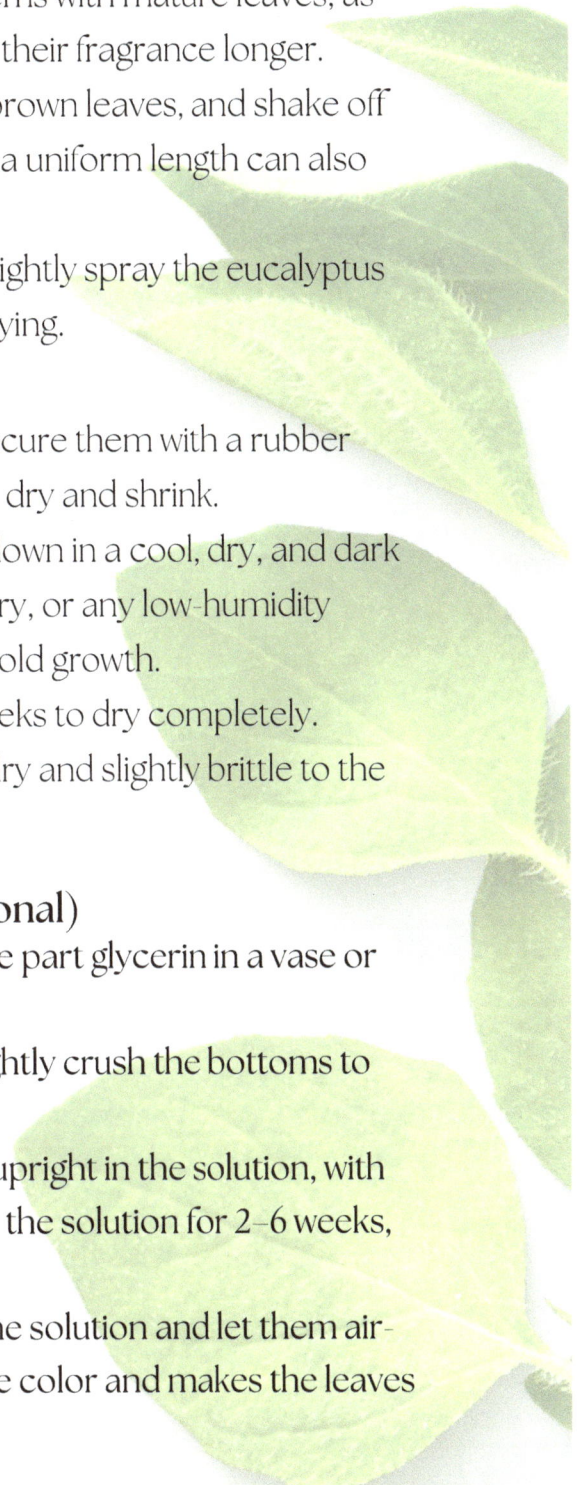

Storing Dried (Spice)

- Storing Dried Eucalyptus: Store dried eucalyptus in an airtight container or a paper bag in a cool, dark place until you're ready to use it. This helps retain the color and fragrance.
- Displaying: Use dried eucalyptus in vases, wreaths, and other arrangements. Avoid placing them in direct sunlight, as it can fade the leaves.
- Refreshing Fragrance: Dried eucalyptus may lose some fragrance over time. To refresh, mist the leaves lightly with diluted eucalyptus essential oil.

Tips for Longevity

- Avoid Moisture: Keep dried eucalyptus away from high-humidity areas to prevent mold and mildew.
- Gentle Handling: Dried eucalyptus is brittle, so handle it carefully to prevent leaves from breaking.
- Rotate Displays: Rotate eucalyptus displays periodically to limit sun exposure, which helps maintain their color.

Seed Collection

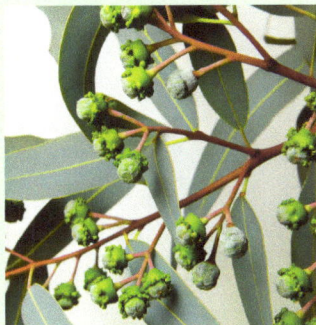

Eucalyptus seeds are small, woody, and found inside the plant's seed capsules, commonly called "gumnuts." These seeds vary slightly in size and shape depending on the species but are typically small, brown, and lightweight. Eucalyptus plants produce seeds as they mature, with seed-bearing typically starting around 3–5 years of age.

When to collect Seeds

- Timing: Collect seeds when the gumnuts are mature, which usually occurs in late summer to autumn. At this stage, the gumnuts will be hard and brown, and they may begin to open slightly, indicating that seeds are ready.
- Maturity: Wait until the gumnuts have turned a light brown to dark brown and feel dry to the touch. Immature gumnuts, which are typically green, will not produce viable seeds.

How to Collect Seeds

- Step 1: Gather the Gumnuts: Using clean pruning shears, cut branches with mature gumnuts attached. It's easiest to clip branches and take them indoors for collection.
- Step 2: Dry the Gumnuts: Place the branches or individual gumnuts in a paper bag or shallow dish and leave them in a warm, dry place for 1–2 weeks. As they dry, the gumnuts will open, releasing seeds.
- Step 3: Extract the Seeds: Shake the bag gently to dislodge any seeds from the gumnuts, or tap the gumnuts over a piece of paper to catch the seeds. Seeds are small and may look like tiny grains or dust particles.
- Step 4: Separate the Seeds: Eucalyptus seeds often come mixed with chaff (small bits of plant material). To separate the seeds, you can lightly blow over them or use a fine sieve to filter out the chaff.

23

Storing Eucalyptus Seeds

- Dry the Seeds Completely: Ensure the seeds are completely dry before storage, as any moisture can lead to mold or spoilage.
- Choose an Airtight Container: Place the seeds in a small, airtight container or a paper envelope if you are storing a large quantity. Label the container with the date and eucalyptus species.
- Cool, Dark Storage: Store the seeds in a cool, dark place, such as a refrigerator, to extend viability. Eucalyptus seeds can remain viable for several years when stored in ideal conditions (approximately 35–40°F or 2–4°C).

Testing Seed Viability

- If you're unsure of seed viability, perform a simple test by placing a few seeds on a damp paper towel and sealing them in a plastic bag. Keep the bag in a warm place, and check for germination over the next 2–3 weeks.

Important Notes on Seed Germination

- Eucalyptus seeds are often sown in late winter or early spring indoors, as they require warm temperatures for germination.
- Plant them shallowly on well-draining seed-starting soil, as they need light exposure for successful sprouting.

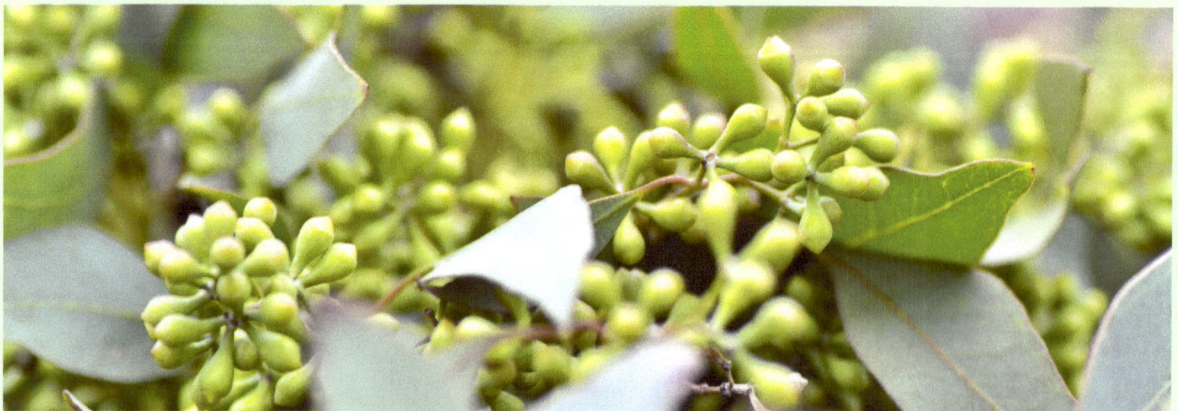

Potential Side Effects
Or Risks

While herbs offer tremendous benefits, they also come with potential side effects or risks, especially when not used judiciously.

Interactions with Medications:

Side Effects: Eucalyptus may interact with certain medications, particularly those processed by the liver, due to compounds that can affect enzyme activity.

Risk Management: Consult a healthcare provider before using eucalyptus if you are on medications, especially drugs metabolized by the liver, to avoid potential interactions.

Skin Irritation and Allergic Reactions

Side Effects: When applied topically, eucalyptus oil can cause skin irritation, redness, or a burning sensation, particularly if used undiluted.

Risk Management: Always dilute eucalyptus oil with a carrier oil (such as coconut or olive oil) before applying it to the skin. Perform a patch test on a small area of skin before full application.

Respiratory Irritation

Side Effects: Eucalyptus oil can cause respiratory irritation in sensitive individuals, particularly young children, as it may cause coughing, wheezing, or shortness of breath if inhaled directly or in large quantities.

Risk Management: Use eucalyptus oil in small amounts and avoid direct inhalation for children under the age of two. Keep diffusers or eucalyptus-infused steam at a moderate level to avoid respiratory discomfort.

Toxicity if Ingested

Side Effects: Eucalyptus oil is toxic if ingested, potentially causing symptoms such as nausea, vomiting, diarrhea, dizziness, and in severe cases, seizures and coma.

Risk Management: Eucalyptus oil should never be ingested. Keep it out of reach of children and pets, as even small amounts can be dangerous if swallowed.

Not Recommended During Pregnancy or for infants

Side Effects: Eucalyptus oil is generally not recommended for use during pregnancy or on infants, as it can be too potent and may pose a risk to fetal development and infant health.

Risk Management: Pregnant and breastfeeding women, as well as caregivers of young children, should avoid using eucalyptus or consult with a healthcare professional for guidance.

Eye and Mucous Membrane Irritation

Side Effects: Eucalyptus oil can irritate the eyes and mucous membranes if it comes into direct contact, causing a burning sensation, watering, or redness.

Risk Management: Avoid applying eucalyptus oil near the eyes, nose, or mouth. If contact occurs, rinse thoroughly with water and seek medical attention if irritation persists.

Dosage and Concentration:

The adage "the dose makes the poison" holds true for herbal medicine. Even beneficial herbs can become harmful in excessive amounts. It's vital to adhere to recommended dosages and to understand the concentration levels, especially with extracts and oils.

When used cautiously and in recommended amounts, eucalyptus can be beneficial; however, it's essential to be aware of these potential risks and consult a healthcare professional when in doubt.

Pests & Disease

IHerb, it is not entirely immune to the challenges posed by pests and diseases.

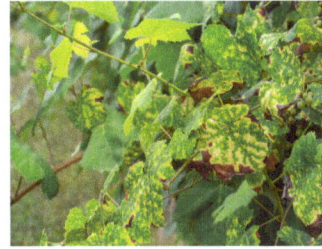

Pests

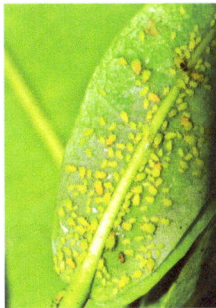

01. Aphids-

These tiny pests sap the life from oregano plants by sucking on the sap of young shoots and leaves, causing them to become distorted and weakened. A strong jet of water can dislodge aphids from your plants. For a more persistent problem, a mild soap solution or neem oil can be applied to affected areas.

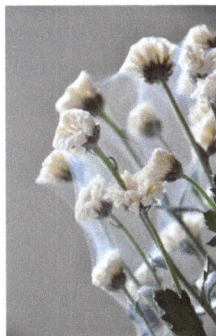

02. Spider Mites

Indicated by fine webbing on the underside of leaves and stunted growth, spider mites thrive in dry conditions. Increase humidity around your plants and use neem oil or a soap solution to treat infestations.

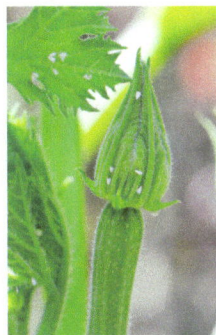

03. Whiteflies

These small, winged pests cluster on the undersides of leaves, sucking sap and weakening the plant. They can be managed by introducing natural predators like ladybugs or by using yellow sticky traps to catch the adults. Neem oil sprays can also reduce whitefly populations.

Diseases

01. Powdery Mildew

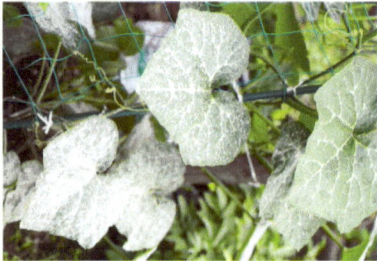

This fungal disease appears as a white powdery coating on leaves and stems, especially during dry, humid conditions. Improve air circulation around your plants and reduce overhead watering to minimize the conditions that favor its spread. Milk spray, a mixture of milk and water, can act as an effective fungicide when applied at the first signs of infection.

02. Root Rot

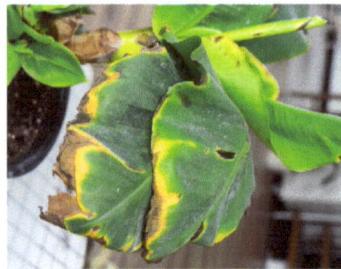

Overwatering is the primary cause of root rot, where the roots of the oregano plant begin to decay, leading to wilting and death. Ensure well-draining soil and moderate watering practices. Infected plants should be removed to prevent the spread of the disease.

03. Botrytis Blight (Gray Mold)

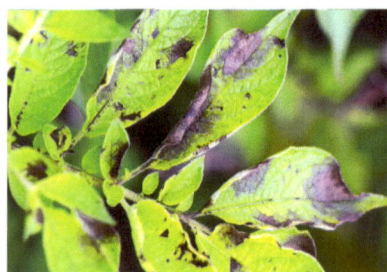

This fungus causes gray, fuzzy mold on leaves, stems, and flowers, thriving in cool, wet conditions. Good air circulation, proper plant spacing, and avoiding wetting the foliage can help prevent botrytis. Remove and destroy infected plant parts at the first sign of disease.

To reduce pests and diseases:
- Remove dead foliage regularly.
- Space out oregano plants for air circulation.
- Plant oregano with tomatoes for health and pest-repellent benefits.
- Attract beneficial insects like ladybugs for pest control and ecological balance.

Universal *Guidelines*

For Adults

- Topical Use: Dilute eucalyptus oil to a 1–3% concentration (about 1 drop per teaspoon of carrier oil) before applying to the skin to avoid irritation.
- Aromatherapy: Use a diffuser with a few drops of eucalyptus oil, limiting exposure to 30–60 minutes in a well-ventilated room to avoid headaches or dizziness.
- Steam Inhalation: Add 1–2 drops of eucalyptus oil to a bowl of hot water for inhalation. Avoid direct contact with the eyes and face and limit use to 5–10 minutes.
- Oral Use: Eucalyptus oil should never be ingested, as it is toxic when consumed.

For Children

- Under 2 Years: Eucalyptus is not recommended for children under the age of 2, as it can cause respiratory distress if inhaled or applied too close to the nose or face.
- 2–10 Years: Avoid using eucalyptus essential oil directly with children. Instead, consider milder essential oils or low-dose eucalyptus-infused products formulated for children. If using a diffuser, place it at a low concentration and limit exposure to 10–15 minutes in a well-ventilated space.
- Topical Use: For children over 10, use highly diluted eucalyptus oil (0.5–1% concentration) if needed, and apply sparingly, avoiding the face and chest area.

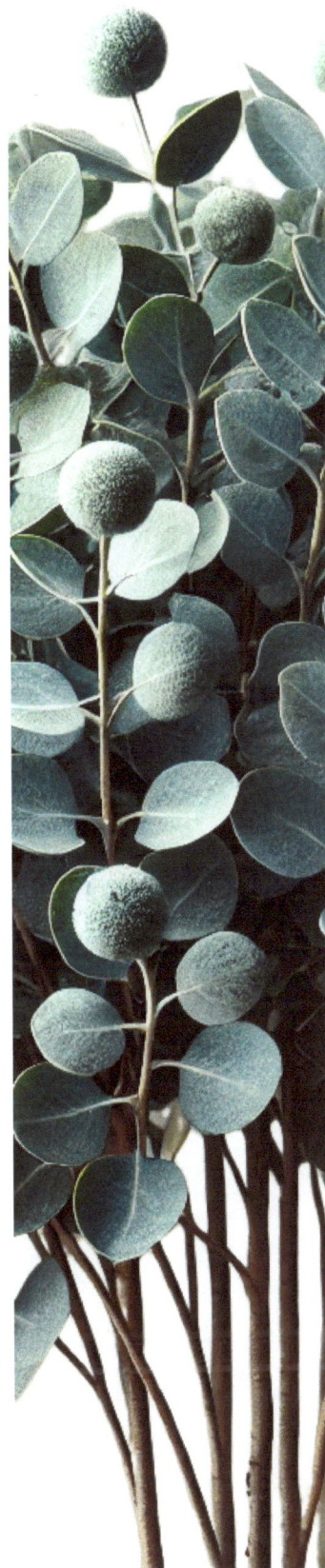

For Pregnant and Breastfeeding Mothers

- General Caution: During pregnancy, it's best to avoid eucalyptus essential oil, especially in the first trimester. Consult a healthcare provider before use.
- Breastfeeding: Avoid using eucalyptus oil on or near the chest area, as the scent could be inhaled by the baby. If needed, use diluted eucalyptus oil (1%) on other areas in moderation and ensure it is thoroughly absorbed to minimize scent transfer.
- Aromatherapy: In well-ventilated spaces, brief exposure in a diffuser (10–15 minutes at a low concentration) may be tolerated, but consult with a healthcare provider to confirm safety.

These guidelines provide a safe framework for using eucalyptus essential oil, but always consult a healthcare professional for advice, especially when using essential oils with children or during pregnancy and breastfeeding.

Moderation is crucial in all aspects, and understanding one's body and its responses is essential. Herbal remedies, though gentle and natural, are potent aids in maintaining health and should be treated with care. It is advisable to seek advice from a healthcare provider or a skilled herbalist, particularly during pregnancy, while breastfeeding, or when tending to young children, to guarantee the safety and effectiveness of herbal therapies.

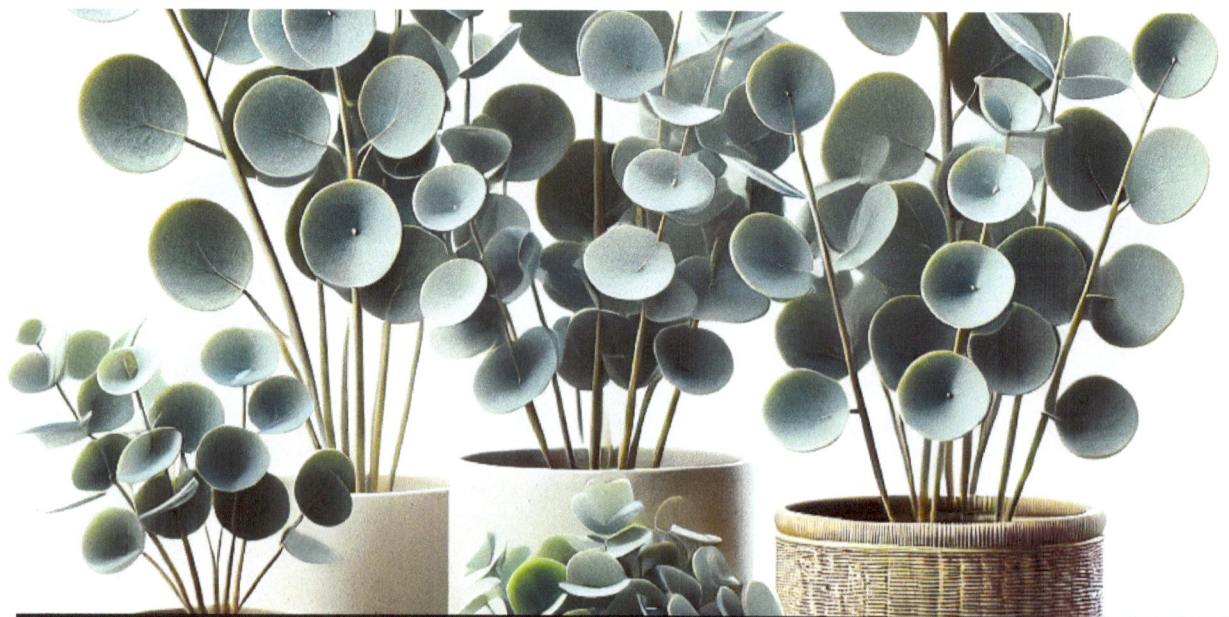

Hydroponics

Hydroponics is a way of growing plants without soil. There are several systems that you can use, with a wide range of cost.

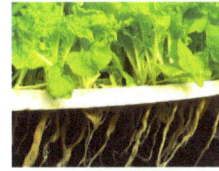

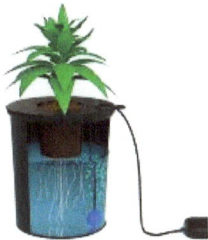

1.DEEP WATER CULTURE (DWC)-PLANT ROOTS ARE SUSPENDED IN A NUTRIENT SOLUTION RESERVOIR. AN AIR PUMP PROVIDES OXYGEN TO THE ROOTS. DWC SYSTEMS ARE RELATIVELY SIMPLE AND INEXPENSIVE TO SET UP, MAKING THEM SUITABLE FOR BEGINNERS. THEY REQUIRE MINIMAL EQUIPMENT AND MAINTENANCE.

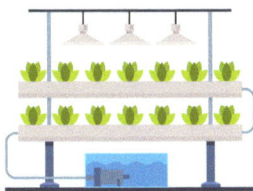

2.NUTRIENT FILM TECHNIQUE (NFT)- INVOLVES A CONTINUOUS FLOW OF NUTRIENT SOLUTION ALONG A SHALLOW, SLOPPING CHANNEL WHERE PLANT ROOTS ARE SUSPENDED. EXCESS SOLUTION IS RECIRCULATED BACK TO THE RESERVOIR. NFT SYSTEMS ARE EFFICIENT IN WATER AND NUTRIENT USAGE BUT MAY BE SLIGHTLY MORE COMPLEX AND EXPENSIVE TO SET UP COMPARED TO DWC SYSTEMS.

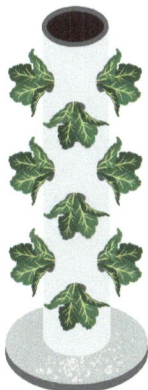

3.DRIP SYSTEM DELIVER NUTRIENT SOLUTION DIRECTLY TO THE PLANT'S ROOT ZONE THROUGH A DRIP EMITTERS OR TUBING. THEY ARE VERSATILE AND CAN BE AUTOMATED FOR PRECISE NUTRIENT DELIVERY. DRIP SYSTEMS CAN VARY IN COMPLEXITY AND COST DEPENDING ON THE SETUP BUT GENERALLY REQUIRE MORE INITIAL INVESTMENT COMPARED TO DWC OR NFT SYSTEMS.

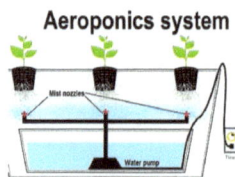

Aeroponics system

4. AEROPONICS SYSTEMS SUSPEND PLANT ROOTS IN THE AIR, AND NUTRIENT SOLUTIONS IS DELIVERED TO THEM AS A FINE MIST OR AEROSOL. THEY ARE HIGHLY EFFICIENT IN WATER AND NUTRIENT USAGE AND CAN PRODUCE RAPID PLANT GROWTH. THEY ARE MORE COMPLEX AND EXPENSIVE TO SET UP AND REQUIRE MORE MAINTENANCE.

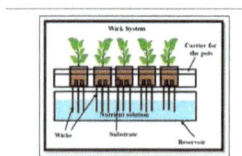

Figure 1: Shows the wick system.

5. THE WICKING SYSTEM USE A WICK TO PASSIVELY TRANSPORT NUTRIENT SOLUTION FROM A RESERVOIR TO THE PLANT ROOTS. THEY ARE SIMPLE AND LOW-COST BUT MAY NOT BE SUITABLE FOR LARGER OR HIGH-WATER DEMAND PLANTS. THIS SYSTEM IS BEST SUITED FOR SMALLER SCALE HOBBYIST SETUPS.

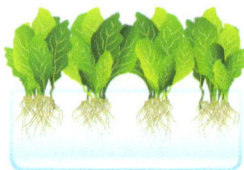

6. THE KRATKY METHOD IS A PASSIVE HYDROPONIC SYSTEM THAT REQUIRES NO ELECTRICITY OR MOVING PARTS. PLANTS ARE PLACED IN A CONTAINER FILLED WITH A NUTRIENT SOLUTION, AND AS THE PLANTS ABSORB THE SOLUTION THE WATER LEVEL DECREASES. THE ROOTS ARE EXPOSED TO BOTH WATER AND AIR, CREATING A BALANCE OF OXYGEN AND NUTRIENTS. THIS METHOD IS STRAIGHT FORWARD AND INEXPENSIVE TO SET UP, MAKING IT AN EXCELLENT CHOICE FOR BEGINNERS OR THOSE WITH LIMITED RESOURCES.

Here is what *We Use*

01. Kratky system

We are currently utilizing two different Kratky Systems:

1. Initially, I opted for dish pans with lids and 2" wide-rim net cups. I am opting for shallow containers to avoid excessive depth because I placed them on shelves and connected lights underneath for more space. , I chose black to minimize algae growth, which has been effective. The wide rim of the net cup secures larger plants like lettuce efficiently, yielding up to 8 plants simultaneously. I stagger the plantings to ensure a continuous harvest, starting them in a tray to establish long roots reaching the water while allowing air access.

2. The second system I am exploring is the bucket Kratky system for growing larger plants such as tomatoes and cucumbers. Seeking sturdier support for trellising, I employ black coloration for algae control. Using pool noodles cut into 1.5" sections with a slit for plant roots, I stack the buckets to create a semi-tower setup. Experimenting with different lighting configurations, I am transitioning to tall stand grow lights on four sides for improved growth. Initially starting tomato plants in a tray to establish water-reaching roots, I have one bucket dedicated to tomatoes and plan to set up another for cucumbers. Adapting the nutrient formula for each plant in individual buckets offers flexibility and customization.

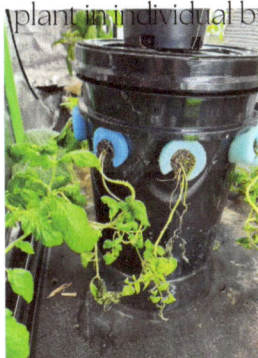

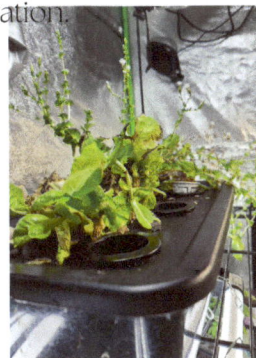

O2. Drip system

My favorite system is the Farmstead, but it costs steeply. It's not a bad price when you use it outside, but I wanted to grow all winter long so I have mine inside, which means I got the one with lights. Love... love... love this system. It only takes a week or two and you can start harvesting lettuce.

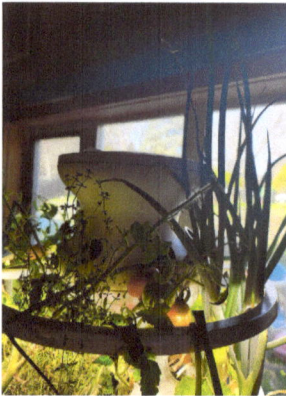

It took a little longer but we have Roma tomato's growing inside during the winter.

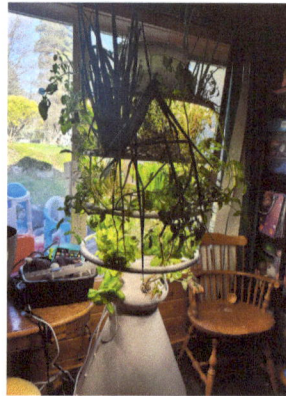

Just look at the growth you can do indoors. I find the system hard to clean, so I will try a different system with a smaller base to see how that works.

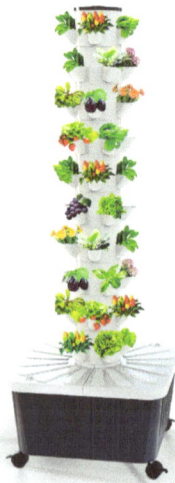

This is the new tower i am using. It works just as good as the farmstand, however you don't get the customer support in growing plants as you do with the Farmstand customer support

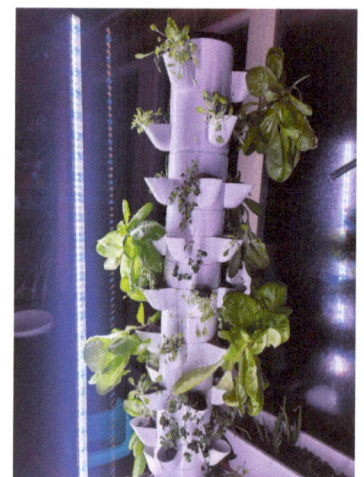

We added tower full spectrum lights to help the growing process, but it is a lot cheaper than the Farmstand. And, its a lot easier to clean

Starters

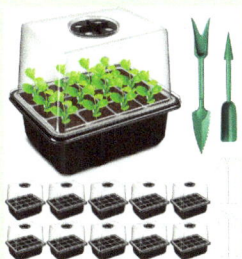

Seed starting trays

https://amzn.to /3xEk6cy

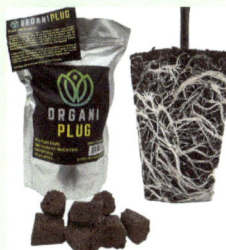

Seed starter Plug

https://amzn.to /4d8eN5m

Heavy Duty Net Pots

https://amzn.to /3W9TVVo

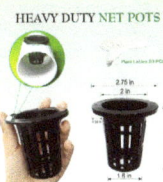

or

Pool Noodles- Use instead of net cups

https://amzn.to /3JsuTJw

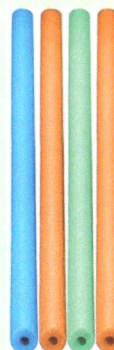

Containers that I use

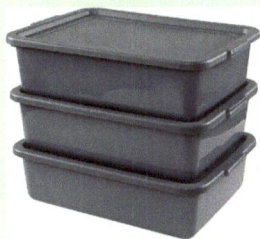

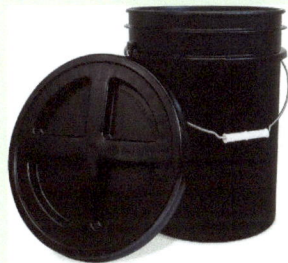

For cutting 2: hole

https://amzn.to /3UpxZnS

Food

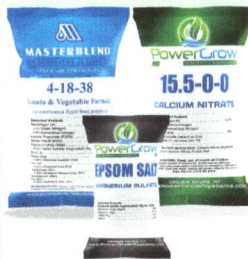

Master Blend Combo Kit

https://amzn.to /3JnPKhj

Dish pan for lettuce and spices

https://amzn.to /4d9bOdd

Sturdy buckets for- tomatoes and cucumbers

https://amzn.to /3U60xBE

Lighting

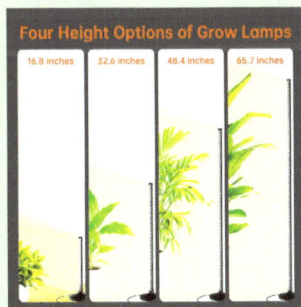

Tall stand lights when you stack your buckets

https://amzn.to /3JnPKhj.

Lighting for starter tray and dish trays

https://amzn.to /3WcHFnj

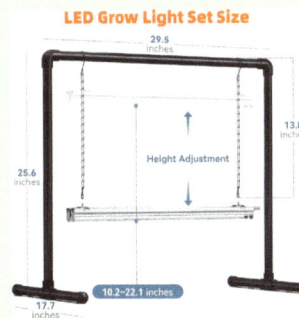

EXTRA'S YOU MAY WANT

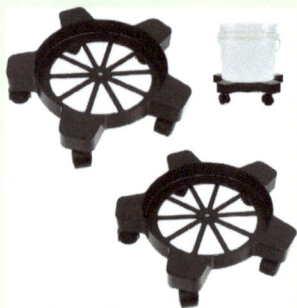

Kennel tray to put everything on. Easy clean up

https://amzn.to/3JsuTJw

Bucket dollies to help you move things around

https://amzn.to/3W761yt

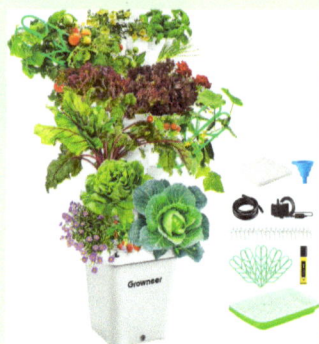

36 plant drip system w/everything including lights

https://amzn.to/49RSLB8

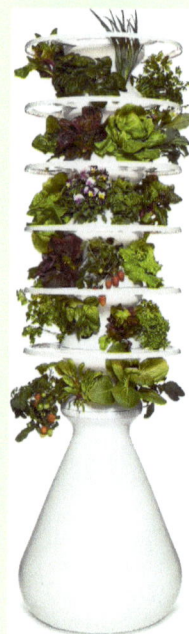

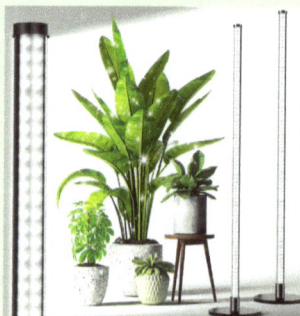

35 plant drip system w/everything no lights

https://amzn.to/3vXdp55

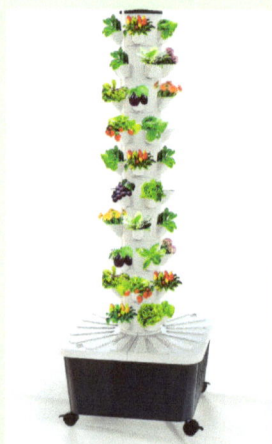

New Lights I found
https://amzn.to/4bp6pfX

New drip tower I am using
https://amzn.to/3W5qQu1

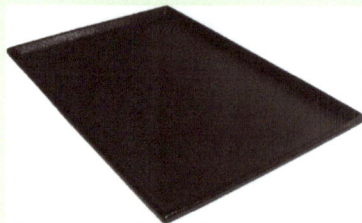

Additional
Considerations

Legal & Ethical

Sustainable Harvesting:
Sustainable practices are paramount whether foraging in the wild or cultivating in gardens. It's essential to harvest in a manner that ensures plants can regenerate, maintaining the health of the ecosystem. This includes taking only what you need and leaving enough behind for the plant to thrive and for wildlife to benefit.

Legal Permissions:
When foraging, be aware of local regulations and property rights. Many areas protect certain species or ecosystems, and foraging without permission can be illegal and harmful to the environment. Please always seek permission from landowners or follow public land guidelines.

Endangered Species:
 Some plants are protected due to their endangered status. Herbalists must stay informed about these species to avoid contributing to their decline. Organizations like United Plant Savers provide resources to identify and protect at-risk plants.

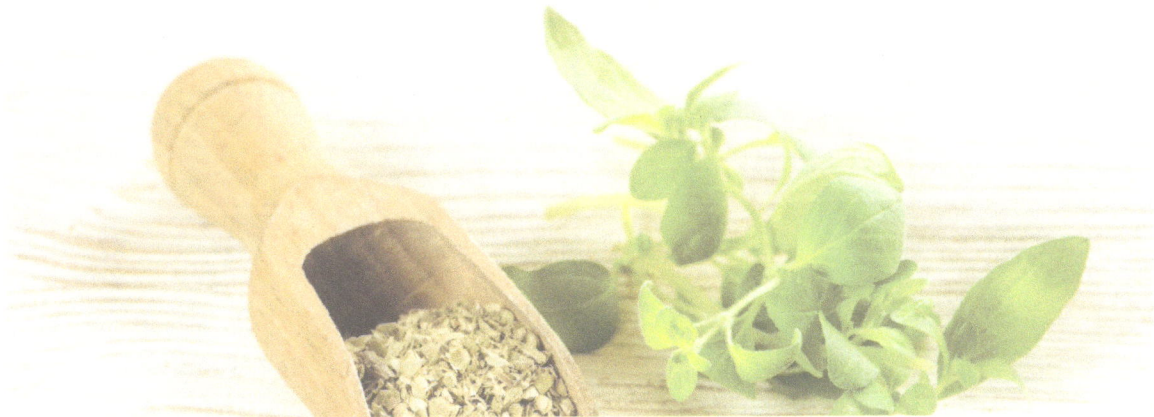

Companion
Planting

spice/herb is a versatile herb that complements many plants when used as a companion. When companion planting, consider the growth habits, sunlight requirements, and soil preferences of each plant to ensure they thrive together. Additionally, interplanting herbs and vegetables can help deter pests, attract beneficial insects, and maximize garden space.

Best Companion plants:

Lavender:
Lavender is drought-tolerant and can handle the same well-drained soil conditions as eucalyptus, making them compatible. Both are aromatic and can create a fragrant garden.

Rosemary:
Like lavender, rosemary thrives in dry, well-drained soil and can withstand the allelopathic compounds in eucalyptus soil. It's also a hardy herb that doesn't require much water.

Sage:
Sage has similar soil and water needs as eucalyptus and can grow well as a companion plant without being affected by allelopathic chemicals.

Thyme:
Another drought-tolerant herb, thyme is a good companion for eucalyptus. Both plants thrive in Mediterranean-type environments with good sunlight and limited water.

Yarrow:
Yarrow is a resilient perennial that tolerates poor soil and dry conditions, so it's often unaffected by eucalyptus compounds.

Many plants are sensitive to eucalyptus and can struggle to thrive when planted nearby due to its allelopathic compounds and its tendency to dominate resources.

Incompatible Plants:

Vegetables (Especially tomatoes, peppers, and other nightshades)

Vegetables generally need richer, moist soil and are highly susceptible to allelopathic chemicals, which can inhibit germination and growth.

Fruit Trees (such as apple and citrus)

These trees require a lot of nutrients and moisture, which eucalyptus may deplete, leaving them nutrient-starved. Additionally, the allelopathic chemicals can hinder their growth.

Annuals and Flowering Plants (like roses, daisies, and marigolds)

Eucalyptus can inhibit the germination and growth of many annuals and flowering plants, which typically need rich, nutrient-dense soil that eucalyptus competes for.

Legumes (bean, peas)

Legumes are sensitive to allelopathy, which can disrupt nitrogen-fixing bacteria in the soil that legumes depend on for growth.

Plants that prefer Moist, Rich soil

Eucalyptus naturally depletes soil moisture and nutrients, making it difficult for moisture-loving plants like ferns, hostas, and hydrangeas to thrive nearby.

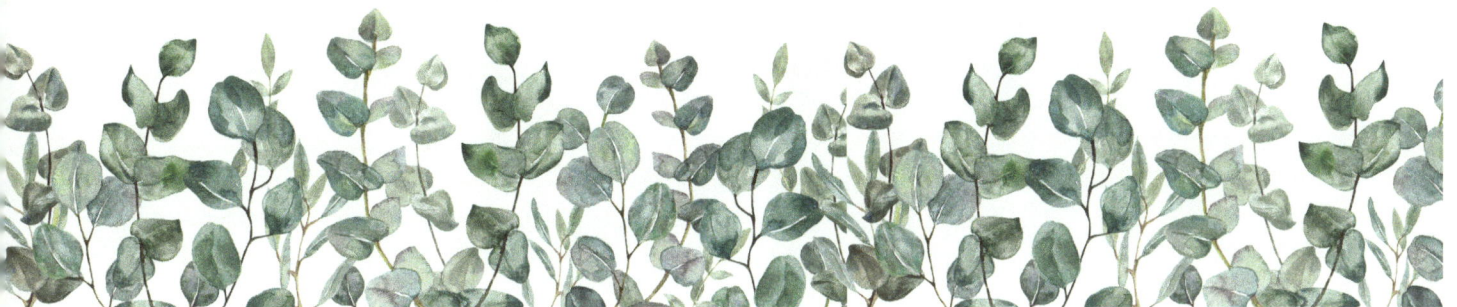

What we learned

Growing eucalyptus at home has been a rewarding journey, though it comes with a few unique challenges. We've learned that eucalyptus thrives with plenty of sunlight, well-drained soil, and regular watering, but it's crucial to avoid waterlogging. These plants do best in a location with good airflow, as stagnant air can make them susceptible to pests like spider mites, aphids, and whiteflies. We've found that misting the plant and ensuring adequate air circulation are effective ways to keep pest activity minimal, helping to maintain a healthy, vibrant plant.

As our eucalyptus plant matures, we're eagerly anticipating its next stages, but it hasn't reached the point of producing seeds yet. This means we haven't been able to collect seeds ourselves. However, we're excited to continue nurturing it and learning more as it grows.

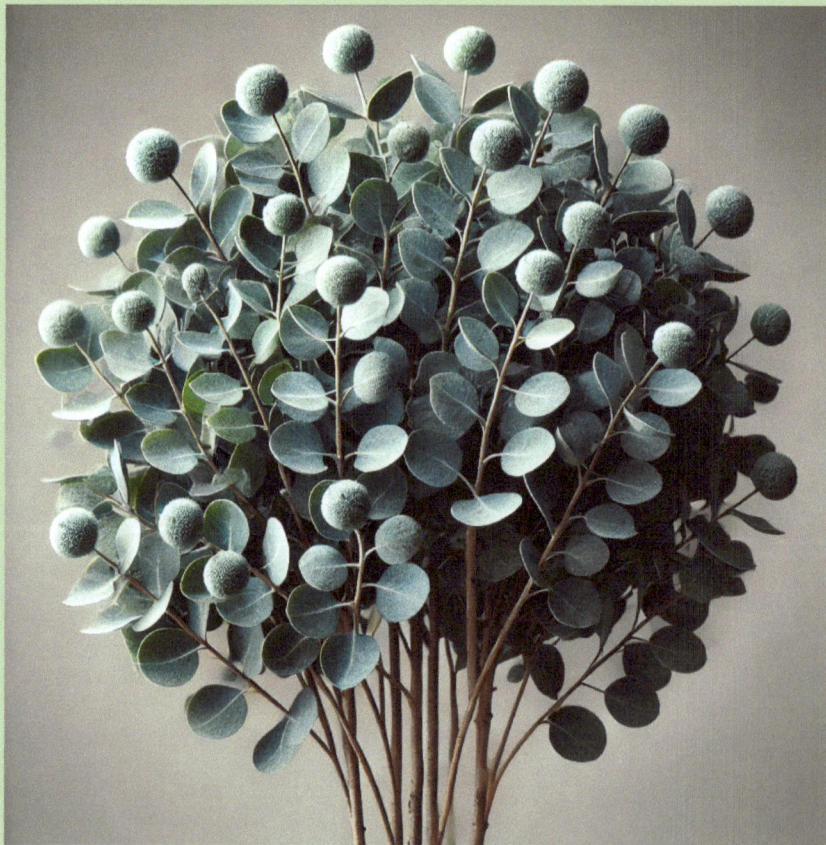

Refrences:

Here's a list of general references and sources commonly used in horticulture, herbalism, and essential oil studies that support information on eucalyptus care, companion planting, medicinal uses, and safety. For specific, highly detailed or scientifically validated information, I would recommend consulting the following types of resources:

Books on Horticulture and Botany:
- The New Sunset Western Garden Book by The Editors of Sunset Magazine: Known for its detailed plant care instructions, including eucalyptus.
- Rodale's Ultimate Encyclopedia of Organic Gardening by Fern Marshall Bradley and Barbara W. Ellis: A reliable guide on organic gardening and plant care.
- The Royal Horticultural Society Encyclopedia of Plants & Flowers: A comprehensive resource on plant species, growing conditions, and plant care.

Essential Oil and Herbalism Resources:
- The Complete Book of Essential Oils and Aromatherapy by Valerie Ann Worwood: Covers safety, applications, and the therapeutic uses of eucalyptus and other oils.
- Medical Herbalism: The Science and Practice of Herbal Medicine by David Hoffmann: An in-depth source on medicinal plants, including eucalyptus, and their health effects.
- The Aromatherapy Encyclopedia: A Concise Guide to Over 385 Plant Oils by Carol Schiller and David Schiller: Provides a breakdown of essential oils and safety guidelines for use.

Peer-Reviewed Journals:
- Journal of Ethnopharmacology: Studies on traditional medicinal uses of eucalyptus.
- Planta Medica: Research on the bioactive compounds of eucalyptus, such as cineole, and their effects.
- American Journal of Essential Oils and Natural Products: Covers safety, medicinal benefits, and applications for essential oils.

Horticultural and Botanical Societies:

Royal Horticultural Society (RHS): Provides extensive plant guides and information on gardening techniques.

American Horticultural Society (AHS): Resources on plant care, companion planting, and soil preparation.

The University of California Agriculture and Natural Resources (UC ANR): Research on allelopathy, eucalyptus planting, and soil interactions.

University Extension Programs:

University of Florida IFAS Extension: Offers specific information on essential oil safety, companion planting, and horticultural practices.

Oregon State University Extension Service: Detailed on eucalyptus species, soil compatibility, and companion planting.

These sources are commonly cited in botanical and herbal contexts, providing trusted information about plant care, medicinal applications, and safe usage guidelines. They're helpful for anyone looking to dive deeper into the details of eucalyptus or other medicinal plants.

Thank You from Simply A Creative Corner

From all of us at Simply A Creative Corner, thank you for purchasing this book and being part of the Empower Your Wellness journey. We truly appreciate your support and hope this resource inspires you on your path to natural healing and healthy living.

We'd Love Your Feedback

Your review means the world to us! Reviews not only support our work but also help others discover resources that may improve their wellness journey.

✦ Leave a review on Amazon:
https://www.amazon.com/stores/Melissa-Poehler/author/B0FNS4WPT9?ref=sr_ntt_srch_lnk_1&qid=1758210089&sr=8-1&isDramIntegrated=true&shoppingPortalEnabled=true&ccs_id=61bd26bb-9338-4d61-8b7e-f428c48f7cec

★ Or share your feedback on Google:
https://g.page/r/CUAi1lOaMhXaEAI/review

Need Assistance?

If you have any questions or need support, please contact us at:
◼ CustomerService@SimplyACreativeCorner.com

Stay Connected

Join our Wellness Corner to stay updated with new releases, wellness tips, and special offers:
https://systeme.io/dashboard/share?hash=75143867cd1b9b84a0e32d5f780ef18941e6&type=campaign

Thank you again for your support—together, we're creating a space where imagination, creativity, and wellness meet.

www.ingramcontent.com/pod-product-compliance
Lightning Source LLC
Chambersburg PA
CBHW060829270326
41931CB00003B/109